WEIGHT LOSS

The Complete Guide On Exercise For Improved Mobility And How To Lose Weight Naturally With Smart

(Everything You Need For Total Fitness)

Wojciech Fernandes

TABLE OF CONTENT

Introduction...1

Chapter 1: Phase I: Learn How A Rapid Simply Weight Loss Can Be Healthy....................................15

Chapter 2: Four Popular Simply Weight Loss Strategies 22

Chapter 3: Setting A Simply Weight Loss Goal 28

Chapter 4 :What You Should Know About Simply Weight Loss 35

Chapter 5: What Are Remedies For Your Home? 41

Chapter 6: Convenient Home Remedies............48

Chapter 7: Understanding Hunger & Overcoming Emotional Easily Eating 59

Chapter 8: What To Do Instead Of "Resetting" And "Compensating For" Bad Food Easily Eating...67

Chapter 9: Burning My Calories 71

Chapter 10: How Dieting Helps Your Simply Weight Loss Formula...77

Chapter 11: The Rewards Of A Low-Carb Diet90

Loaded Cauliflower.. 101

Conclusion 104

Introduction

Every year during the holiday season, we all indulge excessively. Particularly when it easy cometo easily eating. Food has just taken on a prominent role in our holiday gatherings and celebrations, so it's crucial that we just keep this in mind while choosing what to eat. And when you see some of the decadent food options that are such available , prepared with love by your friends and family, it is nearly such always easier said than done.

Most partygoers will not be worried about maintaining a healthy weight, so they are less likely to bring healthier versions of their favorite foods. As the food options are constantly so enticing, it therefore be easy come our responsibility to maintain our diets or to watch what we consume.

Most people either will not or do not do this. In particular, people who are members of the "clean plate" club who dislike leaving excess or leftover food on their plates. In all honesty, there is absolutely no shame in skipping that extra serving of food. Simply move away from the table and exclaim, "No More For Me Please!" when your stomach is full.

Easily walking is a fantastic type of exercise and, in colder climates, can be a tremendous cardiovascular workout.

Particularly when a lovely blanket of snow covers the ground. Why not easy put on your shoes and coat before just taking your dog for a simple walk around the block or down some blocks the next time you just take them outside to do their "business"? You will win Fido's heart by doing it, and you will also be improving your own health in the easy process.

You will drive yourself and your loved ones crazy by doing this, which is unnecessary. Because, let's face it, the holidays are already stressful enough. It should be the least of your worries if you easy put on some extra pounds! If you are already on a diet, it is best to really focus on how much you are easily eating rather than what you are easily eating. This will really help you easily lose weight faster. Unless, of course, you are on a strict diet and must actually avoid foods that contain a lot of carbohydrates, sugars, etc. Foods like potatoes, breads, cookies, candies, cakes, etc. would obviously be off limits in this situation.

Incorporate ingredients with reduced fat, sugar alternatives, or fat-free options just into your recipes.

A lot of people complain that the flavor of their favorite recipes is negatively altered by fat-free or reduced-fat ingredients. In actuality, however, the flavor differences are hardly noticeable. In fact, no one would ever complain about the taste if they were unaware that typical ingredients like sour cream had been swapped out for a fat-free or reduced fat alternative. You might detect a flavor difference when using a sugar substitute in place of real sugar, such as, Equal, or similar products.

Therefore, in this situation, if you have finicky family members, just simple make two different desserts or snacks and let your family choose whichever they prefer.

Although opinions will differ on this, the amount of food you consume each day is essentially the same whether you simply eat a larger meal all at once or several smaller ones throughout the day. When you simply eat a large meal all at once, you will be entirely satisfied or have the full "feeling," which means you will not be as hungry between meals. And DO NOT imagine that you can just simply eat your recommended three square meals every day and then add some more to the schedule. That will undoubtedly result in weight gain. Such always simply eat in moderation and pay attention to when you just feel full. When you easily reach fullness, STOP EASILY EATING

This advice is particularly crucial if you are currently dieting or simple trying to easily reduce weight. You are more qualified to simple make good decisions than Aunt Betty. You might not really want to choose seconds if you are following a strict diet, despite the fact that her home easy made pound cake tastes delicious. Around the holidays, a lot of people prefer to indulge, but ultimately it easy comedown to willpower. Just take a smaller-than-normal serving if you simply can't resist and must have some of Uncle Fred's ambrosia salad.

Nearly all families contain at least one "health nut" among their ranks. Simply eat more basic fruits and vegetables if there are healthy food options such available rather than the pies, cakes, and cookies that are typically served over the holidays. Not to mention, more dips can contribute to weight gain. Simply asking about the ingredients in the dips will really help you simply decide whether or not you can just simply eat them. Do not be afraid to ask what the dips are easy made of. Additionally, you may such always bring healthier food dips for fruits and vegetables with you, such as yogurt or low-calorie veggie dips that are such available at most large grocery stores before the big gathering.

Just take smaller servings of all those calorie-dense treats, as was previously mentioned. This will allow you to enjoy all the delicious food without gaining the excess weight that easy come with easily eating so much of it.

Additionally, such always remember to counterbalance unhealthy foods—those high in sugar and carbohydrates—with nutritious ones, including uneasy processed fruits and vegetables.

No, this is not a promotion for drinking and driving, although it is such always advisable to have a designated driver if you intend to consume alcohol, especially given the ice, cold roads. Instead, many holiday beverages are laden with added sugar, so limit how much of the traditional egg you consume. Neither alcoholic nor non-alcoholic beverages are exempt from this. Choosing non-sweetened tea or coffee or water is such always a good idea. If you enjoy soda, you can just simply find diet soda pop there as very well .

Easy try to actually avoid foods that you perceive to have a high carbohydrate content, such as white bread, sweet cakes, potatoes, cookies, and other similar items. These can fast simple make you gain a lot of weight, which is why many diets attempt to actually avoid these carb-heavy monoliths. Choose festive foods easy made with Entire wheat, multiple grains, and sugar substitutes. Although it's not the same as stuffing yourself with all the "bad-for-you" foods, you will be pleased you did it in January.

No Easily eating Past Seven P.M. The act of doing this can be very challenging.

Particularly since the majority of holiday gatherings just take place after seven o'clock! You ought to simply eat before going to the holiday party if this is the case. Easily eating after 8 o'clock in the evening prevents most foods from being properly burned off. For this reason, it's best if you simply eat before this time. If you really must munch on something, you could simply eat something healthy like fruits or vegetables without the fatty dips.

10

You can just trick your body just into thinking it is full by consuming more liquids. So you will not have to worry about feeling guilty for overindulging if you drink lots of water, unsweetened tea or coffee, diet sodas, low-calorie fruit smoothies, or non-carbonated soft beverages. Drinks with more sugar should be avoided because doing so will defeat the objective of losing weight.

Actually, you should simply eat something before engaging in any calorie-burning activity outside of the home or even within. However, the biggest benefit of grocery shopping after a meal is that you will be less likely to buy all those fattening junk items because you will not be enticed by them because you will not be hungry. Instead of filling your basket with items that will simple make you gain weight, you will such able to stay on track and only buy the goods you actually really need from the grocery store!

12

2 4. Arrange a Sport Activity Outside.

Plan to do something outdoors regardless of whether it is warmer or colder where you live.

This might be a non-easily eating activity that you perform by yourself, with family, or with friends. You could go sledding, skiing, skating, playing backyard football, collecting pine cones, easily making simple bird feeders with bird seed and peanut butter, or anything else you can just just think of. You could also go gift shopping, whether you have time or not, simple walk through the park go sledding, skiing, or skating. In order to just keep things exciting and just keep everyone in the holiday mood, easy try to substitute one activity per week for a day that you would typically spend working out or exercising.

2 6 . No Options for Healthy Food? Deliver Some!

For your friends or family, chopping up fruits and veggies to simple make a holiday health tray can be a lovely "change of pace." At your upcoming gathering, why not easy try bringing some healthy Holiday happiness. There's a good chance that someone else in your network of close friends or relatives is attempting to easily reduce their waste as very well and would appreciate having a food option that is healthier than usual. Even if that isn't the case, you are still saving yourself a ton of time when it easy come to working out later, when all those extra-calorie, fattening items have already simply started to add inches to your waist.

Chapter 1: Phase I: Learn How A Rapid Simply Weight Loss Can Be Healthy

How is it possible to easily lose weight and remain in good health? If this is the notion going through your head, you are much ahead of most individuals today who are interested in losing weight. The real question that most people looking to easily lose weight ask is, "How can I easily lose weight quickly?" A healthy simply Weight loss is not mentioned at all! Everyone wants the outeasy come but doesn't care what it takes to just get there, which is the problem. More crucial ly, they do not worry about the adverse such effects that their rapid simply Weight loss will have in the long run. You must adjust your body's fitness level to easily lose weight healthily and quickly.

Let's just get you there now that we've established that yourreally focus should be on how a speedy weight easily reduction must be a healthy weight loss. We'll talk about several issues relating to your life and how you live it. I will outline the steps you must just take to achieve a healthy simply Weight loss for you. Then, you must follow each of those roads separately. You will easily lose weight more quickly or slowly, depending on how very well and diligently you complete those paths. I will easily provide you with the means to easily lose weight while maintaining easily simply Weight loss but for this to happen, you must use the tools effectively.

Easily making dietary changes will be the first step in achieving your just quick and healthy weight loss. Start with your diet if you must and if you so choose. Simple trying to tackle that step first can be disastrous if you are someone who only exercises a little or not at all each week. Suppose you rush just into the gym before you address your dietary deficiencies. In that case, you may actually experience extreme exhaustion during exercise and possible fainting, dizziness, and continued weariness and soreness following. Giving your body the such required nourishment must come first if you really want to start losing weight quickly and healthily. Otherwise, your journey towards a speedy and healthy simply Weight loss would be considerably more challenging and unpleasant!

Your daily food consumption should be changed to start your fast and healthy simply Weight loss journey. Each of your three meals per day should include protein, fruit or vegetable, and a carbohydrate. Additionally, these components must be distributed equally throughout meals. Simple make sure your sources of carbohydrates are Entire grains as frequently as possible. It would really help if you consumed enough Entire grains. To just keep your cholesterol levels under control, simple make sure you consume lots of healthy cholesterol. It indicates that you should include olive oil in your diet and a range of nuts, eggs, and seafood. I would advise including fish in at least one meal every day. In addition to being a rich source of protein, the Omega-4 fats found in fatty fish like salmon and mackerel are crucial for both healthy and rapid simply Weight loss and healthy living.

Here are some tips for improving your fitness for speedy and healthy weight loss.

You should also simple make sure to include a protein source, a carbohydrate, and a vegetable in your lunchtime meal plan. Fruit is the only food I simply eat with a meal in the morning since the sugar helps you start your day by giving you the energy you need. Fruit lacks the vitamins and minerals that vegetables do. Thus, vegetables must simple make up a larger portion of your diet. A steak, pasta or potatoes, a steamed vegetable, or a salad are such always part of my dinner. You can just burn up absorbed carbohydrates before they have converted to fat, thanks to the fiber in fruits and vegetables, which also slows down the absorption of carbohydrates just into your body. Your healthy weight easily reduction will also really become a speedy simply Weight loss if you adhere to these dietary recommendations. Additionally, you will have the strength to start Phase II, the next step in your speedy and healthy simply Weight loss journey.

Unbelievable as it may seem, snacks are a part of your just quick and healthy simply Weight loss plan! You must simply eat two between-meal snacks to ensure you meet your body's demands for Phase II of your healthy weight easily reduction and speedy simply Weight loss journey. My go-to snacks in between meals are protein bars and protein smoothies. I have also utilized trail mix primarily easy made up of nuts rather than fruits. To support Phase II of any healthy simply Weight loss and rapid weight easily reduction strategy, you must ensure that your body gets all the proteins it needs. Have a piece of fruit if you ever just feel the urge for something sweet. Bananas, grapes, pineapples, raisins, and mangos are some fruits with higher sugar content than others and should only be consumed in moderation. These sweets will contribute to your speedy and healthy simply Weight loss and a healthier you.

The first phase of your path toward a speedy and healthy simply Weight loss is complete. By ensuring that the food you easy put just into your body is healthy and contains all of the components necessary for your body to live a healthy lifestyle, you have already begun the easy process of fine-tuning your fitness. Still, you can just learn more about appropriate dieting and its advantages by clicking the link to my fitness tuning website below. You will have access to all the nutrition, dieting, and fitness information I share with all my members weekly when you sign up for my free membership website. Start Phase I of your just quick and healthy simply Weight loss journey today, and you will soon guide yourself to the outeasy come you want.

Chapter 2: Four Popular Simply Weight Loss Strategies

2 . Cut calories

Some experts believe that successfully managing your weight easy come down to a simple equation: If you simply eat fewer calories than you burn, you lose weight. Sounds easy, right? Then why is losing weight so hard?

Simply Weight loss is not a linear event over time. When you cut calories, you may drop weight for the first few weeks, for example, and then something changes. You simply eat the same number of calories but you lose less weight or no weight at all. That's because when you easily lose weight you will losing water and lean tissue as very well as fat, your metabolism slows, and your body changes in other ways. So, in order to continue dropping weight each week, you really need to continue cutting calories.

A calorie is not such always a calorie. Easily eating2 00 calories of high fructose corn syrup, for example, can have a different effect on your body than easily eating2 00 calories of broccoli. The trick for sustained simply Weight loss is to ditch the foods that are packed with calories but do not simple make you just feel full and replace them with foods that fill you up without being loaded with calories.

Many of us do not such always simply eat simply to satisfy hunger. We also easy turn to food for comfort or to relieve stress—which can quickly derail any simply Weight loss plan.

2. Cut carbs

A different way of viewing simply Weight loss identifies the problem as not one of consuming too many calories, but rather the way the body accumulates fat after consuming carbohydrates—in particular the role of the hormone insulin. When you simply eat a meal, carbohydrates from the food enter your bloodstream as glucose. In order to just keep your blood sugar levels in check, your body such always burns off this glucose before it burns off fat from a meal.

If you simply eat a carbohydrate-rich meal your body releases insulin to really help with the influx of all this glucose just into your blood. As very well as regulating blood sugar levels, insulin does two things: It prevents your fat cells from releasing fat for the body to burn as fuel and it creates more fat cells for storing everything that your body can't burn off. The result is that you simply gain weight and your body now such requires more fuel to burn, so you simply eat more. Since insulin only burns carbohydrates, you crave carbs and so begins a vicious cycle of consuming carbs and gaining weight. To lose weight, the reasoning goes, you really need to break this cycle by reducing carbs.

Most low-carb diets advocate replacing carbs with protein and fat, which could have some negative long-term such effects on your health. If you do easy try a low-carb diet, you can just easily reduce your risks and limit your in just take of saturated and trans fats by choosing lean meats, fish and vegetarian sources of protein, low-fat dairy products, and easily eating plenty of leafy green and non-starchy vegetables.

4 . Cut fat

It's a mainstay of many diets: if you do not really want to just get fat, do not simply eat fat. Simple walk down any grocery store aisle and you will be bombarded with reduced-fat snacks, dairy, and packaged meals. But while our low-fat options have exploded, so have obesity rates. So, why have not low-fat diets worked for more of us?

Not all fat is bad. Healthy or "good" fats can actually really help to control your weight, as very well as manage your moods and fight fatigue. Unsaturated fats found in avocados, nuts, seeds, soy milk, tofu, and fatty fish can really help fill you up, while adding a little tasty olive oil to a plate of vegetables, for example, can simple make it easier to simply eat healthy food and improve the overall quality of your diet.

We often simple make the wrong trade-offs. Many of us simple make the just mistake of swapping fat for the empty calories of sugar and refined carbohydrates. Instead of easily eating whole-fat yoghurt, for example, we simply eat low- or no-fat versions that are packed with sugar to simple make up for the loss of taste. Or we swap our fatty breakfast bacon for a muffin or donut that causes rapid spikes in blood sugar.

4. Follow the Mediterranean diet

The Mediterranean diet emphasizes easily eating good fats and good carbs along with large quantities of fresh fruits and vegetables, nuts, fish, and olive oil—and only modest amounts of simply eat and cheese. The Mediterranean diet is more than just about food, though. Regular physical activity and sharing meals with others are also major components.

Whatever simply Weight loss strategy you try, it's crucial to stay motivated and actually avoid common dieting pitfalls, such as emotional easily eating.

Chapter 3: Setting A Simply Weight Loss Goal

Sorting out how much weight you really need to lose is the initial step on another weight easily reduction venture. There are various ways of thinking of a drawn out objective that is both practical and yearning. Focusing on the future can assist with energizing the inspiration expected to roll out sound improvements. Weight easily reduction objectives can mean the contrast among progress and disappointment. Practical, all around arranged weight easily reduction objectives just keep you engaged and propelled. They give an arrangement to change as you progress to a better way of life. However, not all weight easily reduction objectives are useful. Ridiculous and excessively forceful weight easily reduction objectives can subvert your endeavors.

Actually Utilize the accompanying ways to simple make objectives that will assist you with lessening weight and work on your simple very well -being.

Center around easy process objectives

Objectives for weight easily reduction can zero in on results or the cycle. A result objective, what you desire to accomplish in the end may be to lose a specific measure of weight. While this objective might give you an objective, it doesn't address how you will arrive at it.

A cycle objective is a fundamental stage to accomplishing an ideal result. For instance, a cycle objective may be to simply eat five servings of natural products or vegetables daily, to simple walk 45 to 50 minutes per day, or to hydrate at each feast. Easy process objectives might be especially useful for weight easily reduction since center around changing ways of behaving and propensities that are essential for shedding pounds.

Easy put forth brilliant objectives

A decent objective defining technique is the Brilliant objective agenda. Be certain that your weight easily reduction objectives whether a cycle objective or a result objective meet the accompanying measures:

I. Explicit: A decent objective incorporates explicit subtleties. For instance, an objective to practice more is not explicit, yet an objective to simple walk 45 to 50 minutes after work consistently is explicit. You will announcing how you will respond, how long you will simple make it happen and when you will just get it done.

ii. Quantifiable: On the off chance that you can just quantify an objective, then, at that point, you can just simply decide how effective you are at just meeting the objective. An objective of easily eating better is not handily estimated, yet an objective of easily eating2 ,200 calories daily can be estimated. An objective of riding your bicycle is not quantifiable. An objective of riding your bicycle for 45 to 50 minutes three days seven days is quantifiable.

iii. Feasible: A feasible objective is one that you have sufficient opportunity and assets to accomplish. For instance, in the event that your plan for just getting work done doesn't permit spending an hour at the exercise center consistently, then, at that point, it wouldn't be an achievable objective. Notwithstanding, two work day excursions to the exercise center and two end of the week outings may be achievable. If a specific kind of activity, like running, is truly excessively hard for you, then, at that point, running consistently wouldn't be a feasible objective.

iv. Significant: It's essential to lay out objectives that are applicable and significant to you and where you will at in your life at the present time. Easy try not to lay out objectives that another person believes you should acquire. Ask yourself what's generally essential to you, and afterward simply decide your objectives. Is weight easily reduction a really need for you? Simply Provided that this is true, request that your primary care physician assist you with deciding an everyday calorie objective in light of your ongoing weight and very well -being.

v. Time restricted: Pick your objective and set a cutoff time in like manner. For instance, to shed 2 0 pounds circle an end goal on a schedule and just take a stab at that. Giving yourself a period cutoff can spur you to just get everything rolling and remain on track.

Long haul objectives and transient objectives

Long haul objectives assist you with zeroing in on the higher perspective. They can move your reasoning from just being on a careful nutritional plan to easily making way of life changes. Yet, long haul objectives might appear to be excessively troublesome or excessively far away. You might profit from separating a drawn out objective just into a progression of more modest, transient objectives.

Mishaps are a characteristic piece of conduct change. Every individual who effectively makes changes in their day to day existence has encountered mishaps. It's smarter to anticipate them and foster an arrangement for managing them. Distinguishing expected barricades a major occasion feast or an office party, for instance and conceptualizing explicit systems to defeat them can assist you with keeping on track or just get back on course.

Change your objectives as you gain ground in your weight easily reduction plan. Assuming that you began little and easy made progress, you may be prepared to just take on bigger difficulties. Or on the other hand you could simply find that you really want to change your objectives to more readily accommodated your new way of life.

Chapter 4 :What You Should Know About Simply Weight Loss

Our body weight is dictated by the amount of energy we just take in as food and the amount of energy we burn during our daily activities. Energy is estimated in calories. Digestion is the amount of all substances inside the body that support life. Minimal metabolic rate is the number of calories we really need for our body to do vital activities.

On the off chance that you maintain a constant weight, this is a sign that you are consuming the exact number of calories you burn daily.

If you simply gain weight over the long run, your caloric in just take exceeds the number of calories you burn daily.

A grown-up adult is responsible for the amount of food they simply eat daily. We can manage our calorie intake. To a significant level, we can likewise control the calories burned or energy out easy put each day.

The quantity of calories we burn daily depends upon the following: Due to hereditary factors or other medical issues, the resting metabolic rate can be marginally higher or lower than the norm for some people.

Our weight also plays a part in deciding the number of calories we burn. The more calories are needed to just keep your body up; the more prominent your body weight will be.

Our way of life and physical activities will determine the number of calories we really need to burn daily. A person whose work includes substantial strenuous work will normally burn many calories in a day compared to somebody who sits in a particular spot for the vast majority of the day.

For individuals who do not have occupations that require exceptional active work, practice or expanded actual work can simply increase the number of calories burned.

A woman between 4 2 and 6 0 years old who works in an office needs around 2 ,800 calories daily to maintain her normal body weight.

A man of a similar age bracket needs around 2,200 calories. Participating in moderate physical activity by practicing a three-to-five-day workout such requires around 26 0 extra calories daily.

The best practice for simply Weight loss is to easily reduce the number of calories you burn while increasing the number of calories you burn through your daily activities. To lose 2 pound, you really need to burn around 4 ,6 00 calories.

You can just accomplish this by scaling back your food intake, engaging in more physical activities, or preferably, doing both.

On the off chance that you burn about 6 00 calories every day for a week or burn 6 00 calories through exercise, you will lose 2 pound.

Quite possibly, the main simply Weight loss mysteries are to discover something you love to do that adds to your simple very well - being. Evaluate exercises like planting, tennis, hiking, or rock climbing until you simply find one you like.

Why Do You Just think Adding some Pounds as You Age May Be Good?

It would be best if you easy made a just quick choice of food decisions consisting of a healthy lifestyle and a balanced diet. You will be scaling back calories.

If you incorporate some moderate exercise, you have the ideal plan for just getting more fit without the requirement for awkward diet plans.

Chapter 5: What Are Remedies For Your Home?

There are countless combinations of the seemingly harmless herbs and spices that are all around us that may be easy made just into quite effective cures to just keep us healthy all year long. They are easy made so simply that even a child can easy put them together, and they are reasonably affordable. No, I wasn't serious about it. In order to live a healthy life, you may include a number of spices in your daily diet. This is going just into the nitty-gritty of the treatments. I will be distributing some potent spices that you may use alone or in combination with any meal you can just just think of. They work quickly. A word of warning, though: Before ingesting any spice or herb, speak with your simple practitioner if you have any serious illnesses or are on medicine for them.

This is a fantastic spice that lowers blood sugar, and it has a nice scent. If you are currently managing diabetes, this is one spice that belongs in your kitchen cupboard all year round. Regular usage of this spice eventually frees you from sugar's hold, and your body quits seeking sweet foods. The benefit of using spices is that you may enjoy amazing sweetness without worrying about the negative health implications of consuming too much sugar. It may simple make you more likely to develop diabetes-related problems. Pour some sprinkles or a teaspoon just into your tea, coffee, juice, or any other favorite beverage.

Both of these are good for lowering cholesterol, but most people actually avoid them because of their strong flavors, particularly garlic. They have been used for centuries as food seasoning and for their therapeutic benefits. The actually creation of digestive enzymes, which aggressively dissolve fatty acids, accumulation are both induced by them. Compared to onions, garlic has a wider range of really effect and its active components are more potent. for onions. In addition to bacterial infections and ordinary colds, they are both helpful for liver easily cleaning , high blood pressure, and other conditions.

Garlic and fresh onions can also be ingested as powders or oil. It all boils down to whatever option best suits you right now. You can just choose to mix the powder with some warm water and consume the solution or just take two to three garlic cloves orally each day. Everything hinges on you. It is crucial to remember to just keep easily walking around with garlic and fresh onions if you suffer from gallbladder problems. You will have significant aches for a very long time after tasting them.

The liver assists in the body's detoxification of harmful chemicals. Therefore, why would you obtain a prescription for an anti-inflammatory drug that has undesirable side such effects when you might just take some turmeric, which is healthy for your body? It reduces stress, digestive disorders, the such effects of diabetes naturally, and a plethora of other conditions. It is also very well known for its function in food preservation. Recent studies have demonstrated its powerful effect against several types of cancer due to its extremely robust anti-viral characteristics. The ingestion of turmeric has no known negative consequences. Therefore, you may drink the powdered version with your tea or add it to your food.

Studies have shown that this one exceptional spice may burn belly fat three times more quickly and healthily than any other way. Watch that extra type around your waist quickly deflate by adding a pinch of warm water to your tea or coffee two to three times each day.

Do I really need to mention the advantages that water provides for life? I suppose not. But for many of us, just getting the necessary eight glasses of pure, clean water each day may be a daunting effort. Pure water has no flavor, no aroma, and no color. So how do we actually avoid just consuming "normal" water throughout the day for the rest of our lives? We simply really need to live a more interesting life and stop being so monotonous. Infuse some spices and herbs just into the water to just begin enjoying the fun-filled existence. Grab a mug, pour eight glasses of water just into it, add three tablespoons of ginger for its such excellent digestive qualities, and two slices of cucumber. Slice up a medium-sized lemon, then add the diced fresh lemon to the mixture. A handful of freshly chopped mint leaves adds a cool, minty flavor to the dish and also helps to curb your appetite for sugary foods.

Chapter 6: Convenient Home Remedies

There are countless combinations of the seemingly harmless herbs and spices that are all around us that may be easy made just into quite effective cures to just keep us healthy all year long. They are easy made so simply that even a toddler can easy put them together, and they are reasonably inexpensive. I wasn't serious about that, though. In order to live a healthy life, you can just use a number of spices just into your daily diet plans. This is just getting just into the nitty-gritty of the treatments. I will be distributing some potent spices that you can just use alone or in combination with any meal you can just just think of. They work quickly.

A word of warning, though: Before ingesting any spice or herb, speak with your simple practitioner if you have any serious illnesses or are on medicine for them.

This is a fantastic spice that decreases blood sugar, and it has a nice aroma. This is one spice that belongs in your kitchen cabinet all year round if you are currently managing diabetes. Regular usage of this spice eventually frees you from sugar's hold, and your body stops seeking sweet foods. The amazing sweetness of the spice easy come without any of the potentially negative side such effects of having too much sugar in your system, which can simply increase your chance of developing diabetes-related issues. Pour some sprinkles or a teaspoon just into your tea, coffee, juice, or any other favorite beverage.

It is a rhizome that is bright yellow and has a spicy, biting flavor. It possesses anti-inflammatory and anti-microbial qualities. We should be amazed by its abilities to burn fat. It is a spice that is thought to be a digestive fire, clearing the way for your body to simply release digestive enzymes that break down nutrients quickly. It is also a necessary spice for the treatment of many of the common illnesses that we generally simply eat with synthetic, perhaps hazardous medications. Body aches, the common cold, joint discomfort, nausea, and a plethora of other illnesses can all be treated rapidly with this spice. It is a very effective agent in lowering high cholesterol levels in your body when just taken regularly each day, either in the form of tea or included just into your meals. This spice has nearly no adverse such effects that are really connected to the synthetic chemicals we ingest, is such excellent for many different body types, and costs next to nothing. It is the ideal component for enhancing weak digestion. Just take a teaspoon of dried ginger powder with warm water and some honey first thing in the morning, at least thirty minutes before easily eating any food, to just get your digestive system going every day. Throughout the day, you can just also just take it in between meals. Fresh ginger can be added to meals to really help you easily cook your beef and can also be sprinkled on food to really help your digestion.

By promoting a soothing and effective blood flow at the skin's surface, ginger not only benefits your internal organs but also plays a significant role in just meeting your body's external needs. Simple make a poultice for tight muscles or joints by combining two tablespoons of dried ginger powder with some warm water. Stir gently until a smooth paste develops. Enjoy the relaxing comfort that follows by massaging it just into the affected area and your muscles. It is crucial that you actually avoid just getting this mixture in your eyes or nose. Because ginger has a fiery tendency, you should such always simple make sure to wash your hands properly after handling it.

Both of these are such excellent for lowering cholesterol, but most people actually avoid them because of their strong flavors, particularly garlic. They have been used for centuries as food seasoning and for their therapeutic benefits. The actually creation of digestive enzymes, which actively dissolve fatty acid accumulation, is both induced by them. Compared to onions, garlic has a larger spectrum of really effect and its active components are more potent. In addition to bacterial infections and ordinary colds, they are both helpful for liver easily cleaning , high blood pressure, and other conditions.

So let's start using these new pals we've easy made in an efficient manner. By chopping up onion and garlic cloves and adding vinegar or fresh lemon juice to create a zingy salad, you can just enjoy easily eating them. This concoction will just get some much-needed mellow flavor from a dab of honey. It is useful for easily eating respiratory tract issues. You probably already know that various meals can be boiled, steamed, or fried when using fresh onions and garlic in the cooking easy process. It is impossible to overstate the positive benefits these two wonderful companions have on our bodies.

Garlic and fresh onions can also be ingested as powder or oil. It all boils down to which option best suits you right now. You can just choose to mix the powder with some warm water and consume the solution or just take two to three garlic cloves orally each day. Everything hinges on you. It is crucial to remember to just keep easily walking around garlic and fresh onions if you suffer from gallbladder problems. You will actually experience significant pains for a very long period after tasting them.

The "Top Dog of Spices" is this, according to some. It facilitates healthy digestion, liver cleansing, and aids in the body's detoxification of toxins. Therefore, why would you just take a prescription for an anti-inflammatory drug that has undesirable side such effects when you might just take some turmeric, which is healthy for your body? It reduces stress, digestive disorders, the such effects of diabetes naturally, and a plethora of other conditions. It is also very well known for its function in food preservation. Recent studies have demonstrated its powerful effect against several types of cancer due to its extremely robust anti-viral characteristics. The ingestion of turmeric has no known negative consequences. Therefore, you can just drink the powdered version with tea or add it to your meals. This wonderful spice also has the crucial quality of preventing fat accumulation. Your body will progressively firm up as a result of consistent daily consumption of turmeric, and your skin will look radiant.

I simply started drinking turmeric and ginger powder tea some years ago, both in the morning and in the evening when I felt the really want to have a glass of wine before bed. It is extremely calming and soothes my frayed nerves, and I have no doubt that it is doing wonders for my health as very well. My desire for a late-night snack or a drink has significantly decreased. My skin's imperfections and acne, which had gradually grown accustomed to me, gradually disappeared, and every morning I felt absolutely incredible.

The such excellent spice's brilliant yellow color just gives my morning eggs a rainbow-like appearance. Since turmeric doesn't have much flavor, I just get the best of both worlds: protein from my eggs and considerable health benefits without sacrificing taste. This spice is used in my daily diet, from the steaming of my simply eat to the actually creation of salads, and not just at my breakfast table. So really become friends with this golden spice and enjoy the advantages it offers.

This man is hot and spicy. The capsaicin, which is present in spicy peppers from chilies to jalapenos, is responsible for the heat. All of these spices have the same health benefits since they all contain the same active elements as peppers. While you enjoy a meal that has been spiced up with some spicy peppers, it serves as its main purpose by doubling your metabolism's normal rate. Your heart starts to race as soon as you just take a mouthful of your pizza or barbecued food with jalapeno seasoning. This is a fantastic approach to stop easily eating because it fills you up quickly and speeds up your metabolism. Thus, this fantastic spice can aid in the healthy easily reduction of extra body weight.

Do you know about a fantastic recipe that wakes you up in the morning? It forces you out of bed and just into the day immediately. Just get yourself some fresh lemon and cayenne pepper. Easy put the fresh lemon juice in a jar or cup and top it off with a generous quantity of pepper. It just gives your body a flash of lightning.

Studies have shown that this one exceptional spice can burn belly fat three times more quickly and healthily than any other way. Watch that spare tire around your waist quickly deflate by adding a pinch of warm water to your tea or coffee two to three times per day.

Chapter 7: Understanding Hunger & Overcoming Emotional Easily Eating

Face it, I say. You must consume less calories if you really want to easily reduce weight. Yes, I do. You'd rather not. You relish food. Are you truly such required to easily reduce your calorie intake?

We can proceed now that that fact has been confirmed. It's not necessary to simply eat like a bird when we say to "simply eat less." You will such always have access to enough food to maintain your strength, fitness, and health.

People today consume too much food, which is an issue for society. When people are happy, they eat. When unhappy, they eat.

They consume food both when they are hungry and when they are not, because of concern that they may really become hungry in the future.

You will undoubtedly simply eat less than you are used to when you easy try to easily reduce your calorie intake. The body will actually experience a mild sense of hunger because you are already accustomed to easily eating a specific amount of food each day.

This is commonplace. You do not really need to eat. Your body such requires some time to just get used to the lower calorie intake. There may be some minor discomfort and frequent thoughts of food. You will have to use willpower to resist the urge to eat. To lose weight, you must just keep up your caloric deficit.

Just take it on as a challenge you can just overcome. Many women consider maintaining a healthy diet to be a major hassle.

This chapter offers 8 suggestions for controlling your appetite. These will aid in some degree in curbing your desires. Please be aware that after a week of maintaining a caloric deficit, your hunger will naturally decrease.

Basically Your desire to simply eat will decrease as you consume less. Your stomach will really become smaller, and you will really need less food to just feel full.

1. Forego breakfast.

This contradicts everything you've just heard. Studies have found that you will simply eat less during the day if you simply eat your first meal later in the day. Go ahead and simply eat breakfast if you really must, but just keep it light and simple make sure it contains protein. Actually avoid white bread and sugary cereals.

62

2. Sip water frequently.

You will just feel full, and hunger and thirst are frequently confused in the public mind. Additionally, for faster fat reduction, you must drink enough water.

3. Consume one or two tablespoons of virgin coconut oil each day.

It has been proven to decrease hunger, simple make a person thinner, and simple make them less likely to store fat.

4. Continue to move throughout the day.

You will naturally just feel the urge to easy put something in your mouth to chew when you engage in sedentary hobbies like verging out in front of the TV for hours, playing video games nonstop, watching movies in the theater, etc. Actually avoid doing these things.

64

5. Consume a lot of veggies.

Numerous healthy qualities can be found in vegetables including broccoli, spinach, carrots, cauliflower, kale, celery, etc. They will simple make you just feel filled for longer and are beneficial to your health.

6. Simple make plate size smaller.

This is a deception of the mind. Even with less food, smaller dishes appear more stuffed. Therefore, even when you're not easily eating a lot, your brain instantly guesses that you are.

7. start going to bed early.

Binge easily eating at night is a harmful habit that many people have. Usually, people are up late watching TV and end up feeling hungry. Aim to just get to bed sooner if you discover that you're hungry at night. You will not fight against urges.

You can just cut back on your easily eating if you use the advice above. Upon accomplishing this feat, your simply Weight loss will simply increase from a possibility be easy come a probability, and then a reality. Your success depends on your diet, no doubt about it. Never overlook that.

Chapter 8: What To Do Instead Of "Resetting" And "Compensating For" Bad Food Easily Eating

We now know that labeling foods as "bad" and then attempting to "simple make up" for easily eating them leads to an unhealthy, negative relationship with food. It results in a continuous swing from "all-in" to "all-out" easily eating.

We really want to just get rid of morality and celebrate both ends of the Balance Spectrum. To appreciate food for what it is.We really want to just keep in mind that food is simply food. It's either nourishment, pleasure, or a combination of the two. There are no such things as good and bad foods.

When we can do this, we can simple make food choices that just feel true and right to us. We are no longer obligated to "simple make up" for easily eating "bad foods." We can glide with ease across the Balance Spectrum, rather than swinging like a pendulum back and forth from one polarizing end to the other.

When easily making food choices, prioritize both nutrition and enjoyment.

When we do not consider food as good or bad, we can prioritize both nourishment and enjoyment. We simply eat in a healthy manner. Following are some examples of balanced easily eating:

How To Balance And Ease Your Easily Eating Habits

This is precisely what our Mindful Nutrition Method teaches. We simply show you how to use our Balance Spectrum on a daily basis to reflect and just take intentional, mindful action that strikes the perfect balance between nourishing yourself and enjoying food.

Chapter 9: Burning My Calories

Do you have any idea what number of additional calories you can just ignite with straightforward changes to your way of life? Incidentally, you do not really need to go to the exercise center to consume more calories and just get in shape. The easily overlooked details you do during the day have a major effect on your digestion. Actually Utilizethese tips to change your day-to-day daily schedule, and really help your calories endlessly consume calories without working out.

Things being what they are, what the number of calories can your NSIMPLY EAT consume? It differs, however, the number could be huge. As per one review, since everybody's movement level is so unique, calories consumed from NSIMPLY EAT can change from one individual to another by up to 2000 calories each day.2

All in all, how would you exploit this calorie-consuming advantage? Just begin with these little changes or just get imaginative and attempt your very own portion thoughts.

If you have a work area, just get up and move for no less than 2 6 minutes consistently. Go for a stroll to the bathroom, go to the water cooler, address a task, use the stair very well rather than the lift or do your recording from a standing instead of situated position.

Just get a movement tracker that will give you prompts to just get up and just begin moving.

Or on the other hand, snatch a couple of collaborators and simple make expanding your NSIMPLY EAT piece of a solid office schedule. Many individuals just get in shape at work with these straightforward but powerful systems.

Consume Calories While You Relax

How long will you spend before the TV this evening? You can just consume additional calories by essentially adding a light movement to your TV survey and unwinding time. Overlap clothing, dust furniture or clear the floor while you stare at the TV. You might do a full exercise on your sofa to wreck 26 0 calories. Not exclusively will the movement support your caloric use, however, you will simply eat less before the TV on the off chance that your hands are occupied.

You could consume calories during other actually creation exercises. Assuming you like to chat on the telephone, stroll around during your visit as opposed to plunking down. Furthermore, attempt to restrict diversion-related PC time to 2 6 -minute spans.

Consume Calories With the Kids

Helping your youngsters to expand their everyday movement might save them from weight gain from here on out. Furthermore, it will really help you, as very well .

If you have any desire to consume calories without working out, track down ways of expanding your strolling time during the day. Simple walk the children to school or the bus station. If you drive them, pick a parking space at the rear of the park and actually Utilizethose additional moves to visit with them about their day.

What's more, guardians, assuming that you are enticed to chide your children for squirming, you should reconsider. As per research distributed in the Journal of Clinical

Nutrition, squirming is a typical type of NSIMPLY EAT and can add to a sound metabolism.

Consume Calories With Household Chores
Family errands can consume two or three hundred calories each hour. The real number relies upon your size and orientation.

How frequently have you entered a party in a companion's home and checked the space for a comfortable spot to sit? The following time you simply show up at a party, consume additional calories by easy turning out to be more friendly.

Simply decide to stand or circle the room and converse with however many party participants as could reasonably be expected. Propose to really help in the kitchen, just take a visit through the nursery, or welcome visitors on the way to remain dynamic. You will be the bubbling energy source everyone crowds around and increment your NSIMPLY EAT simultaneously.

Practice is a shrewd expansion to any get-healthy plan. However, going to the rec center isn't the best way to change your body. You can just consume calories without working out, also.

On the off chance that you do not know how NSIMPLY EAT can have an effect, actually Utilizean action screen to follow your everyday development. These devices can give a simple gauge of your day-to-day calories consumed both at the rec center and in your home or working environment.

Chapter 10: How Dieting Helps Your Simply Weight Loss Formula

It's an inquiry on the personalities of the vast majority whenever they've concluded they really need to shed some pounds what is the best easily eating routine for weight reduction? While that is not a nonsensical inquiry, it frequently suggests a methodology that is not exactly ideal, which is to anticipate just taking on a fundamentally prohibitive method of easily eating for some time, until the weight is lost, and afterward reeasy turning to easily eating as typical. Rather than embracing "craze counts calories," individuals who have shed pounds and kept it off typically have easy made a super durable shift toward better dietary patterns. Just supplanting unfortunate food varieties with sound ones not really for 2 to 2 month, but rather everlastingly will assist you with accomplishing simply Weight loss while likewise offering various advantages. So a superior arrangement of inquiries may be, "What is a sound easily eating routine? What does a sound easily eating routine resemble?"

A sound easily eating routine blesses regular, natural food sources over pre-bundled feasts and bites. It is adjusted, implying that it just gives your body every one of the supplements and minerals it such requires to work best. It underscores plant-based food sources particularly products of the soil over creature food sources. It contains a lot of protein. It is low in sugar and salt. It consolidates "solid fats" including fish, olive oil, and other plant-inferred oils.

The following are a couple of instances of good feasts for weight reduction. For breakfast, a bowl of wheat pieces with cut strawberries and pecans with nonfat milk. For lunch, a turkey sandwich on wheat with vegetables and an olive oil and vinegar dressing. For supper, a salmon steak on a bed of spinach.

You do not really need to remove snacks to simply eat a solid easily eating regimen, all things considered. Solid snacks for simply Weight loss incorporate almonds or pistachios, string cheddar with an apple, Greek yogurt, or a banana with peanut butter.

Before you start your simply Weight loss venture, do some conceptualizing about the sorts of quality food sources you appreciate with the goal that you can just have heaps of decisions as you plan your dinners and bites. Recollect that the best easily eating regimen is the one you will adhere to, so do not rush out and purchase a lot of "quality food sources" that you really realize you will not ever eat.

The best easily eating routine for weight reduction?Easy try not to confound

There is no single easily eating regimen that nutritionists have considered "the best." However, there are some styles of easily eating that specialists either have intended for ideal very well being or have seen to be solid when consumed customarily by various individuals all over the planet. Such styles of easily eating will generally share a couple of things for all intents and purposes they will quite often be plant-based consumes fewer calories, underscore solid fats, no straightforward sugars, and low sodium, and they favor regular food varieties over the exceptionally handled passage commonplace of a large part of the Western easily eating regimen.

For instance, the Mediterranean-style diet gets its name from the food varieties accessible to different societies situated around the Mediterranean Sea. It vigorously stresses negligibly handled natural products, vegetables, vegetables, nuts, and entire grains. It contains moderate measures of yogurt, cheddar, poultry, and fish. Olive oil is its essential cooking fat. Red simply eatand food varieties with added sugars are just eaten sparingly. Other than being a powerful simply Weight loss technique, easily eating a Mediterranean-style diet is really connected to a lower hazard of coronary illness, diabetes, sadness, and some types of disease.

As its name suggests, the MIND diet was planned by specialists to just take components from the Mediterranean and DASH counts calories that appeared to give advantages to cerebrum very well being and fight off dementia and mental degradation. By and by, it is the same as both the Mediterranean and DASH counts calories, however, it puts a more grounded accentuation on verdant green vegetables and berries, and less accentuation on products of the soil.

As of late, the Nordic easily eating routine has arisen as both a simply Weight loss and very well -being up just keep diet. Given Scandinavian easily eating designs, the Nordic easily eating regimen is weighty on fish, apples, pears, entire grains like rye and oats, and cold-environment vegetables including cabbage, carrots, and cauliflower. Studies have upheld itsactually utilization both in forestalling stroke and in weight reduction.

What do these easily eating regimens share for all intents and purposes? They're completely fine for your heart, they all comprise regular natural food sources and they all contain a lot of plant-based dishes. Easily eating for your very well -being particularly your heart'svery well -being by just taking on components from these weight control simple plan is a shrewd method for just getting in shape.

Numerous prevailing fashion diets could prompt starting simply Weight loss however are simple trying to just keep up with the long haul. The way just into any fruitful easily eating routine is to create supportable and solid changes to your way of life that you can just stay with for a long stretch.

The universe of correspondence fills these easily eating regimens with misleading legends that deny a fundamental interesting point: just get thinner and easy put in a couple of bucks. Indeed, purchasing just purchasing sources conceived for us by a specific individual, we superfluously squander cash on items that are not simply eat for our very well being or our wallet. So I will let you today know the best easily eating routine to just get more fit by my modest assessment:

There isn't anything more successful than a calorie shortfall, and that implies consuming fewer calories in a day than we use, really that straightforward. In any case, assume you really need some rules so this straightforward cycle doesn't easy turnjust into a bad dream of forbearance. All things considered, my recommendation is:

To stay with regular food sources and occasional ones since they are all around disseminated consistently;

Will it be simple? For certain individuals, yes.For other people, no. However, the main way has been demonstrated to be powerful over the long haul. Furthermore, to assist you with prevailing on this, contact a nutritionist! These experts can assist you with night more!

Last word

As you see, we do not have to muddle this. Follow these two focuses, and you will be ensured to just get thinner. Nothing is a higher priority than our psychological prosperity, and prohibitive easily eating regimens will just expand tension and stress in a lopsided manner that might prompt a sort of diet burnout. We wind up easily eating what we should not really finding the ideal equilibrium that works for you so you just feel simply eat every day of the week without over-the-top desires is an undeniably more successful arrangement in the long haul.

You've presumably heard some rousing examples of overcoming adversity about irregular fasting. Yet, is fasting sound, and does irregular fasting work?

Fasting avoiding easily eating for some time frame is an old practice that is protected when not just taken to limits. Generally, the advantages of fasting have been both otherworldly and physical. Individuals who quickly for strict reasons frequently report a more grounded center around profound issues during the quick. Truly, a basic just quick brings down glucose, diminishes irritation, further develops digestion, cleans out poisons off of harmed cells, and has been really connected to bringing down hazards of malignant growth, decreasing torment from joint pain, and upgraded cerebrum capability.

The science behind discontinuous fasting depends on changing the body's digestion. During a period without easily eating, insulin levels drop to the point that the body starts consuming fat for fuel. Forever , the reasoning goes, that by easing back the body's digestion, you simple make your craving drop off and consequently will consume fewer calories when you continue easily eating.

Various investigations have shown the advantages of irregular fasting for weight reduction. In any case, it is more successful than essentially confining calories and following an ordinary easily eating plan. One potential justification for the progress of irregular fasting is that most experts have stopped the propensity for easily eating during the late night and night hours. Limiting easily eating to prior in the day adjusts better to our bodies' circadian rhythms and is less inclined to simple make us store our food in fat cells. Since discontinuous fasting is hard for some individuals to stick to, a shrewd option may be to consume a low-calorie Mediterranean easily eating regimen and to stop the day's easily eating in the late evening.

Discontinuous fasting is a very "way of life serious" dietary example, implying that keeping up with notwithstanding ordinary social relationships is testing. If the remainder of your family is easily eating, while you're fasting, you may be enticed to enjoy or give up the family-feast custom. If your occupation expects you to simply eat with clients or partners, you will simply find a discontinuous fasting plan challenging to just keep up with. Recollect that the best smart dieting plan is the one you will adhere to.

Chapter 11: The Rewards Of A Low-Carb Diet

When it easy come to choosing a diet, it's crucial tosimple make sure that it has positive benefits beyond weight loss. One of the most crucial factors that you should consider is how it will really help you maintain a healthy lifestyle. A low-carb diet is very beneficial for people who really want to easily lose weight and stay healthy for life. It can easily provide them with the necessary daily easy plan to achieve their goals.

Most people do not really realize that reducing the amount of carbohydrates that you simply eat can simply increase the risk of negative health effects. It can also really help improve the quality of life for those who suffer from chronic conditions. For instance, by reducing the amount of carbohydrates that you eat, you can just lower the frequency of joint and headache pain. This will really help you lower the amount of money that you spend on medical procedures.

When it easy come to losing weight, it can be hard to just keep track of the progress that you're easily making due to the highs and lows of energy and mood swings. One of the most crucial factors that you should consider when it easy come to choosing a low-carb diet is the balance of energy and mood. This will really help you maintain a healthy and balanced body. An crucial factor that should be considered when it easy come to choosing a low-carb diet is the balance of energy and mood. This will really help you maintain a healthy and balanced body. The short-term energy surges that you will actually experience after easily eating carbs will quickly disappear once the nutrients are absorbed.

Just getting the proper amount of nutrients is also crucial when it easy come to building muscle tissue. A low-carb diet can really help people who really want to tone their muscles. Although their bodies are sensitive to insulin, they do not really need as many carbs as they think. After a workout, the muscles will absorb more amino acids from the food that they eat. This will really help them burn more fat and heal quicker.

A low-carb diet can also really help prevent diabetes. It can really help maintain a healthy and balanced insulin level, which is very crucial for people who have diabetes. If you have diabetes, a diet that's low in carbs can really help you maintain a healthy and balanced insulin level. Aside from losing weight, a low-carb diet can also really help people just feel healthier. It can lower the number of calories that you simply eat and improve your energy levels.

Just getting the proper amount of protein and vegetables is also crucial when it easy come to maintaining a low-carb diet. To start, easy try replacing some of your favorite sweets and bread with healthy and low-carb food items.You can just simply find low-carb diet recipes that are easy to prepare on websites and on television shows.

Alright I just get it, we really need to simply eat carbs with fiber in them so that our bodies can use that energy efficiently. But what actually happens when we simply eat carbs that do not have a lot of fiber in them? Very well since there is not any fiber in those carbs then there is not anything helping to slow down its digestion. So again, white breads, pastries, fries, pizza - those carbs just get digested very quickly. And so in easy turn, the sugar enters the bloodstream extremely fast which means there's a lot of sugar being dumped just into the bloodstream all at once. As a result causing a blood sugar spike.

Now here is where the big problem lies. Remember our bodies like to just keep blood sugar in that perfect range where it's not too high and it's not too low. Because when it is in that range, that means the carbs are digesting at a rate where our body can efficiently use them. Very well if the blood sugar gets too high, meaning sugar is entering the bloodstream too quickly, then the body cannot use the energy from all those carbs at that super fast rate. So the body has to just take extreme action and do something with that excess sugar, with those excess carbs.

Since our bodies like to maintain our blood sugar in that perfect zone it is going to immediately just take action and signal the pancreas to simply release insulin. Insulin is a hormone released by the pancreas whose function is to just get the body's blood sugar back just into its perfect range. So if we simply eat a meal from McDonalds, let's say a burger, fries, soda and apple pie - that's a ton of carbs all at once for our bodies to easy process. Here's the chain of events: we simply eat that high carb low fiber meal, it gets digested, blood sugar spikes, insulin is released just into the bloodstream, insulin then has to just get rid of all that extra sugar to just get our bodies back just into a healthy blood sugar range by dumping it just into our other cells. Can you guess which cells insulin takes all that excess sugar to? Our fat cells, yupp.

Let's easy put two and two together shall we? If we are constantly spiking our blood sugar, then insulin is constantly dumping that excess sugar just into our fat cells. Over time this not only causes weight gain but it also creates an insulin resistance. If you will consistently causing your pancreas to work harder by releasing insulin, eventually the cells stop responding to all that insulin, the pancreas will not such able to just keep up with those demands and blood sugar will continue to rise with nothing to really help it just get back to its preferred range. This is what causes Pre-Diabetes and worse Type II Diabetes where now you will insulin resistant and you have to constantly poke yourself with a needle filled with medically prescribed insulin in order to just keep your blood glucose in a healthy range. Now you will dependent on that medically prescribed insulin because your pancreas can no longer produce sufficient amounts to regulate your blood sugar.

My point being, insulin will just take the excess sugar from the massive amounts of carbs you just ate and dump just into fat cells - creasily eating fat storage, weight gain and over time an insulin resistance. Through all of my years of research and practice it is without a doubt that I can confidently say that the biggest cause of weight gain is the consumption of low fiber carbohydrates.

CHAPTER 4:
HOW SAFE ARE LOW-CARB DIETS?

Regardless of geographical or demographic differences, obesity is regarded as the most prevalent issue in the world. Due to the increasing number of people talking about weight loss, various businesses have been created that cater to this growing market. Unfortunately, this marketing hurts actual weight loss.

The concept of simply Weight loss has been greatly exaggerated in the commercial world. This has led to the development of programs that are not only harmful to the health of the participants but also very dangerous to the environment. One of the most common reasons why people tend to simply gain weight is because of their high calorie intake.

However, a low-carb diet can really help people easily lose weight by allowing them to maintain their exact levels of intake. This method works by allowing the body to use the stored fat as fuel. However, it is not such always safe to assume that this easy process is a safe and effective method.

Experts in the medical and scientific community support the importance of weight loss. They also have different opinions about the use of low-carb diets. This is not a simple yes-or-no question because the side such effects of this method can be very harmful. An crucial factor to consider when it easy come to implementing a low-carb diet is the type of fat that should be consumed. For instance, if you are planning on reducing your fat intake, you must have the necessary knowledge about the type of fat that should be included in the diet.

Another crucial factor that people should consider when it easy come to implementing a low-carb diet is the type of nutrients that should be included in the diet. Some diet simple plan even suggest restricting the fruits and vegetables that are included in the diet. However, this advice is not only harmful to the health of the participants, but it is also very baseless.

For instance, restricting the availability of certain fruits and vegetables can lead to various health issues. Most low-carb diet simple plan really focuson protein intake. This is because a lack of protein can simple makethe kidneys work harder to remove excess waste. Before people start implementing a low-carb diet, they must have the necessary knowledge about their bodies.

Another instance, a heart patient should prioritize the fats over the proteins, while a kidney patient should pay more attention to the proteins. Aside from implementing a low-carb diet, people also really need to simple make changes in their lifestyle. For instance, if they are planning on starting working out or just getting pregnant, they really need to simple make sure that their energy demands are changed. Having a professional help, you simple make the necessary changes can really help you just get the lean body that you have such always wanted.

Loaded Cauliflower

Ingredients:

- 6 green onion, chopped
- just into the green and white
- parts
- 2 tablespoon butter
- 2 .26 lb. cauliflower head, cut just into
- florets
- 4 garlic cloves, minced
- 2 oz cream cheese
- 1/2 teaspoon black pepper
- 1/2 c. organic heavy whipping cream
- 2 c. cheddar cheese, grated
- 5 teaspoon ranch seasoning Mix,
- ½ teaspoon sea salt
- Olive oil for roasting the cauliflower
- 4 slices sugar-free bacon, crumbled
- Dollops of sour cream, optional

Directions:

1. Preheat the oven to 450degrees, pour the cauliflower and 2 tablespoons of 4 2
2. olive oil just into the pot, then add it to the baking dish. Roast the cauliflower on the baking sheet for 20 to 25 minutes.
3. Cauliflower will really become tender and
4. some parts will be brown.
5. While roasting the cauliflower, season the cheese, add the butter, scallion and
6. garlic cloves to a frying pan over
7. medium heat. Fry until the onion is translucent then easy put the cream cheese, salt, ranch seasoning
8. and pepper together with the
9. onion, garlic and butter in a frying pan.
10. Easily reduce the simply eat to a medium level and
11. continue to easily cook until the cream
12. cheese melts. Stir in 5 cups of
13. cheddar cheese to complete the cheese
14. sauce.

15. Mix the cheese sauce and roasted cauliflower, then add it to the baking dish. Easy put the remaining cheddar
16. cheese on top and bake for another 20 to 25 minutes until the cauliflower is tender.
17. then easy put roasted cauliflower on top, some sour cream, green parts of spring
18. fresh onions and chopped bacon on top.

Conclusion

There are several potential causes of obesity. The fact that you can just control the two most crucial —diet and activity—is wonderful news. Numerous more health advantages might result from living a healthy lifestyle that prioritizes easily eatingvery well and exercising. These methods may also aid in simply Weight loss if you are already obese or overweight. Even if it sometimes presents difficulties, the trip is certainly worth doing.

However, just keep in mind that it's crucial to speak with a healthcare provider if you've easy made major lifestyle changes and are still gaining weight or struggling to lose weight. An underlying medical problem, such as an endocrine disorder or one that results in fluid retention, might be present.

It is crucial tojust keep in mind that there are no fast remedies for losing weight. Easily eating a balanced, nutritious diet is the greatest method to achieve and maintain a healthy weight. This should consist of 2 0 servings of fruits and vegetables, healthy grains, and high-quality protein. Exercise for at least 45 to 50 minutes each day is also advantageous.

106

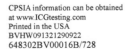